Intermittent Fasting for Women

How to Eat What You Want and Still Lose Weight While on a Budget

By

Beatrice Anahata

been derived from various sources. Please consult a licensed professional before attempting any techniques outlined in this book.

By reading this document, the reader agrees that under no circumstances are is the author responsible for any losses, direct or indirect, which are incurred as a result of the use of information contained within this document, including, but not limited to, —errors, omissions, or inaccuracies.

Table of Contents

Introduction

Congratulations on grabbing your copy of *Intermittent Fasting for Women: How to Eat What You Want and Still Lose Weight While on a Budget* and thank you for doing so.

The following chapters will discuss the different types of safe intermittent fasting methods, and how to shop on even the slimmest of budgets. It is full of tips on how to eat healthy, exercise, and still save money while making the lifestyle change to intermittent fasting.

There are plenty of books on this subject on the market, thanks again for choosing this one! Every effort was made to ensure it is full of as much useful information as possible, please enjoy!

Chapter 1: Fasting Can Be Your New Normal

The word fasting does not exactly conjure happy thoughts, you might even feel your stomach growling just thinking about going a long time without food. However, that is not really the case; there is no reason you have to go long periods without food. Instead, there are many different methods of fasting for you to choose from that will allow you to find the one that works best for both your lifestyle and your body. As you read about the different methods, think about which one jumps out at you, the one that you think would fit into your life the best. Also rule out which ones you think definitely wouldn't. No two people are alike and if something sounds absolutely terrible to you, chances are it would be. So be realistic. There are many options to choose from, and remember, it is a lifestyle change and some discomfort is only natural.

It is important to know that the female body does react different in ways than a male's body. That is because there are different types of hormones that are active in a woman's body to make sure all systems are behaving and performing properly. The biggest and first thing the body will sacrifice when it feels as though it is in starvation mode is the reproductive system. You don't want this to happen, so it is important to follow the rules of the fasting methods and not push yourself too hard. You want to safely reduce your caloric intake, not hurt yourself. That is why you want to do this safely and in a way that works with your body instead of against it. Remember, this is not a one size-fits-all type of deal, you are in complete control of how you choose to fast.

Intermittent fasting simply means not consuming food for a predetermined period of time, generally between twelve to 48 hours. Many people call this time the "fasting period", and what you do consume during this time is completely up to you. For instance, some people decide to only drink water during their fasting period, while others add black coffee, herbal tea, or even different types of bone broth. What you do decide to consume during this time is your choice; even if someone you know only drinks water, do not feel like you need to do the same. Everyone is different, and you might be happier if you get to enjoy your morning cup of coffee, or if you would like to drink green tea throughout the day. At the end of the day, this is your fast, your body, and the goal of fasting is not to make you feel miserable.

Some people think that you are not able to exercise while intermittent fasting, but this is simply not true. There are going to be days and times when you are able to eat normally, and this also means you can and should exercise normally as well. Should you choose the method that requires you to fast for a full 24-hour period, or drastically reduce your caloric intake, don't choose those days to exercise too hard. Instead, do lighter exercises on these days and don't force yourself to work too hard to the point of exhaustion or pain.

How Fasting Works

After you eat, the body spends hours processing the food and burns what it can of the meal you ate. This means that your body has all of it; easily available fuel to burn to create energy. This means that your body will use the food that you just ate to burn instead of stored fat. As you probably know, in order to lose weight, you need to burn fat stores, not just the food you just consumed. This holds especially true if you ate a lot of carbohydrates and sugars because the body will burn sugar before anything else. Keep that in mind when you are eating, because even though you have gone hours during your fasting time, you do not want to overdo it when you do eat by eating too many carbohydrates and sugars.

Of course, this does not mean that you need to give up everything you love. As a matter of fact, nearly everything is fine in moderation. When you are fasting, your body has not only burned off your last meal, but it has also moved passed that and started to burn off fat stores, which is the key to losing weight. Some people think that, because they fast, they are going to want to eat twice as much when they do eat, but that is not the case. Granted, sometimes your meals are going to be a little larger than the meals you had before you began fasting, but your body will adjust rather quickly, and you will find that you are full even though you have skipped a meal or two.

Fasting Methods

Crescendo Method: This is a great introduction to fasting because it does not affect your hormones and does not have a negative impact on your body. Basically, it does not shock the body's systems. The secret to this method of fasting is the schedule and shorter fasting hours. The Crescendo method can also be tailored to fit into your lifestyle, for instance, you fast two or three non-consecutive days each week. On these days, you will fast for between twelve and sixteen hours, again you get to choose the amount of hours that work for you. For instance, sixteen hours might seem too long and, but fourteen fits better into your lifestyle and does not make you miserable.

These hours do not need to be during peak hours of activity either. Most people choose to stop eating at 7:00 p.m. and fast until 9:00 a.m. the next morning. This is just one example. Beginning your fast at 5:00 p.m. and ending it at 7:00 a.m. might work better for you and so on. Just make sure you choose non-consecutive days and that you begin and end your fast at the same times on each of these days every week.

Continuity is important because you want your body to adjust, and constantly changing the times is not going to help your body, it will only set you back.

The Crescendo method is also effective because you will be fasting for shorter, less frequent periods of time, while still decreasing your general caloric intake, but preventing the body from going into starvation mode. Keep in mind that this is still a different way of eating, and in the beginning your body is probably going to go through a rebellious phase. This does not mean it is in starvation mode, it is just something new that it needs to adjust to, and it will given time and patience.

16/8 Method: This is one of the most common methods of fasting. It is not a dip your into fasting method though, it is a bit more intense than the Crescendo method, but it does yield results. The 16/8 method means that the 24-hour day is broken up into eight hours and sixteen hours. The eight hours are the eating window and the 16 hours are the fasting period. This is not done only certain days of the week, but every day, which is what makes it a bit more intense. However, it is easy to schedule since you don't have to think about the days of the week, you know which times you are allowed to eat each and every day.

Again, this is not a one-time-fits all method. You get to choose which eight hours to eat and when to fast.

One of the most common times is eating from noon to 8:00 p.m., but this might not work for everyone. You can change the times around to suit your lifestyle. You might want to make breakfast a priority, so starting your eating period at 8:00 a.m. and beginning your fasting period at 4:00 p.m., this might seem difficult, but it is up to you. This method can also work for people who work night shifts, which is one the reasons it is so popular since there is so much freedom to choose the fasting and eating times. So, for those people who work throughout the night, their eating times can begin at midnight and end at 8:00 a.m. so it fits into their lifestyle, since they will do their sleeping during the daytime hours. Other diets do not take into the consideration the large amount of people who live a less traditional time-based lifestyle because their sleeping happens mostly during the daylight hours.

Now, once again, even though it is called the 16/8 method, it does not have to be that way. You can even change the times if you choose to, shortening or lengthening by a couple of hours if you need to. Some people choose to do 18/6, meaning they fast for eighteen hours and eat for six, or even 20/4. Do what works for you, just make sure you are continuous in your efforts and give your body time to adjust. The body will not go into starvation mode in sixteen hours, especially since traditionally, nearly half or more of those hours are spent sleeping. Your body is capable of so much, and this is a great way to drastically decrease your caloric intake and burn body fat. Fasting is meant to be a way for the body to burn fat stores, and with this method it most certainly will.

Eat-Stop-Eat Method: This is also a rather common method of fasting because it is used by so many people. It is safe for both men and women and has gained popularity since it can be tailored to fit into so many schedules and lifestyles. This is the one method that does not necessarily require you to stick to such a strict schedule since you can choose the amount of days you want to fast. They do have to be non-consecutive days, but they do not need to be same days each week. With the eat-stop-eat method you simply do not eat for a 24-hour period, two to three days per week.

This is definitely a more intense form of intermittent fasting simply because the body is going to go 24 hours without food, and for some it can incredibly difficult to adjust to. However, the body will still not enter starvation mode from a 24-hour fast. That does not mean that this method is necessarily the easiest either, since the body is accustomed to eating each day. That is why with this fasting method, it is encouraged to drink water and other beverages throughout the day. Many people who practice this method do not restrict their beverage intake on fasting days, enjoying cups of tea, black coffee, and even the very occasional diet soda.

Even though some people do choose to fast three times a week, two is the recommended amount. The other thing that sets this type of fasting method apart from the others is that people generally refer to their eating days as 'feasting days', not because they get to eat whatever they want in moderation. It is not a good idea for anyone to go overboard with sugars and carbohydrates, and this includes those practicing intermittent fasting, but you can still indulge within reason. The recommended amount of calories for a woman to intake on feasting days is around 2,000 which is more than most traditional diets will allow. Fasting for two 24-hour periods during the week will reduce your caloric intake by around twenty percent, while still allowing you to eat the foods you love.

5:2 Method: This is also called, the 'fast diet'. It is another common form of intermittent fasting for women, but it might not fit into everyone's schedule and it does require counting calories, and for some people that is just not what they are looking for in a fast. Unlike with the other methods, the numbers in the name of the method do not refer to hours, but instead the days of the week. Five days of the week are regular eating days, again, remember that your diet still needs to be rather healthy in order to see results. The other two days of the week, again not two consecutive days, you will consume only 500 to 600 calories.

This means that you will have to pay close attention to the number of calories you are eating on the restricting days. Basically, you want to restrict your caloric intake to a quarter of your traditional intake two days of the week. That is why so many people do prefer this method because there are no full days without eating. A good example of this is to restrict on Mondays and Thursdays, while eating normally throughout the rest of the week. Make sure to eat three small meals on the restricting days and keep close track that each meal not exceed the daily limit when added together. On average, on restricting days meals should be around 200 calories each.

As with the other methods, you can switch the days of the week you want to restrict, just make sure they are the same each week. You can also change the amount of days too, if you choose to. For instance, instead of 5:2, maybe you want to do 4:3, eating normally for four days and restricting for three. Do not exceed more than this though, because this crosses over into dangerous territory and you might end up doing more harm than good, with the most common result being moodiness and weight gain.

Once You Have Made Your Decision

So, you have chosen your method of intermittent fasting, now it's time to actually begin your fast. This is when things can get rather difficult because your body is adjusting to this new way of eating. The first two weeks of any intermittent fasting are difficult, keep that in mind. You might feel like giving up, you might feel like eating anything in site, but this feeling will pass, it just takes time. Remember, there was a time when your body couldn't even consume solid foods, but it learned how. This is the same thing. You need to give your body time to relearn and adjust.

In the beginning you might experience some unfortunate, but common side-effects such as dizziness, irritability, headaches, and even insomnia. Remember, these will pass as they are all part of the process. Your body is learning to burn fat stores and not to simply depend on the meals you have recently consumed since you are going to be either drastically restricting calories or going longer periods of time without consuming calories.

If after two weeks these symptoms persist or get worse, take a step back and reevaluate your chosen method. You might need to choose a different method. Not everyone's body is the same and some fasting methods work better for some and not for others. It might be a simple solution such as switching the fasting days to the days where you are typically less active, or moving around the eating hours to fit into your daily schedule a bit better. So, before giving up, try moving the times around and see how your body reacts to that.

Also, don't forget that you can drink some bone broth or tea to help. This is especially important if you choose to fast for 24-hour periods as this is a difficult method to adjust to. Many people find that drinking tea or coffee also helps them because it makes them feel as though they are not depriving their body of everything. Remember, sometimes the ritual of making coffee or tea is just as important as the consumption of it and depriving your body and brain of that ritual it has come to rely on so heavily can have detrimental effects. So, allow yourself that daily indulgence, just skip the cream and sugar on the fasting days. Some people have a tendency to compare themselves to others, try your best not to do this. Yes, some people can do the eat-stop-eat method and happily consume only water for a 24-hour period, but if you are not one of those people, that's fine. Don't force yourself to be miserable. This is more than just a diet, it is a lifestyle change, and it is not intended to make your life more stressful or to cause you long lasting discomfort.

It is normal for a lifestyle change to be difficult, so listening to your body is important. That's why there are so many different, but still effective methods to choose from. Each person is different, and the way in which someone responds to a certain fast is also going to be different. The people who are most successful at intermittent fasting are the ones who understand that it might take some trial and error. There is no shame in making changes if your first, second, or even third attempt did not work for you.

If you commit to the lifestyle change and make the changes that make it easier for you, you will increase the chances of success. Just like with anything else in life, there is no such thing as instant change or gratification. It is going to take some time for you to see changes, but it will happen. When you are practicing intermittent fasting, you are cutting calories which means you will lose weight. Some of the other added benefits to intermittent fasting include an increase in energy, mental clarity, and even saving money.

When you are first starting your chosen method, it is best to sit down and work out a schedule. You can do this on your phone, a calendar, or even just a piece of paper. Having something in front of you that breaks down the days so you know when your eating and fasting periods are broken down week by week for the entire month, will help put things into perspective. Doing this will also help you schedule personal events and obligations as necessary, because temptation is going to happen, this is especially difficult in the beginning. Sometimes the best thing to do is avoid this until you are more comfortable in your fasting method and your body has adjusted. Doing this will also help increase your chances of success and make the transition to intermittent fasting easier.

Chapter 2: Eat, Just Know When to Do It

Even though you are fasting, you are still going to eat. However, that does not mean that during eating periods you get to eat whatever you want all the time. Just like in everyday life, everything is technically fine, but in moderation. If you fill your body with nothing but over processed foods and sugar during eating periods, you are probably going to gain weight, but this would be true with or without intermittent fasting. The rules for gaining or losing weight do not change. Intermittent fasting is a lifestyle change that is supposed to make it easier to cut out calories because you are eating only during specific times.

For those people who already eat a pretty healthy diet, one that is not full of empty carbohydrates and sugars, this is not going to be too much of a shock to them. However, if you are a fast food, carbohydrate, and sugar lover and that is mostly what your diet consists of, then you are going to need to make more of a lifestyle change than others. You can still eat these things, just learn to limit your intake. Remember, during your eating periods, you still only want to consume around 2,000 calories. It is very easy to go over that limit if you are not paying some attention to what you are eating. The method that requires the most attention to caloric intake is the 5:2 method because for two days you are not to exceed 600 calories at most. This is a low amount of calories and without careful calorie counting, it can be very easy to overdo it and surpass that limit. For some people, they don't want to have to count calories that closely, and that is perfectly okay, that just means that this method is not for them.

Let's assume you chose to go on the 16/8 method, and you have your daily schedule set up. That means each day you have eight hours to eat your 2,000 calories. How you choose to consume those calories is completely up to you. Some people prefer to have the three traditional meals with no snacks in between. Others would rather have two larger meals with some light snacking in between their meals. Just remember that you are not trying to make up for lost calories by eating more calories since you went so long without eating. Don't worry, your body is not going into starvation mode and will actually adjust to this new schedule probably better and easier than you imagined. Again, the first two weeks are going to be the worst and after that, for many people, it simply becomes their regular way of eating and they simply don't think about it anymore.

Dealing with Cravings

For those who have a sweet tooth, you do not have to give up sugar, just make sure to factor it into the allotted amount of calories during your eating periods.

Some people will avoid sugar altogether for the majority of their eating periods, and then one day a week indulge in a rich dessert. Others prefer to have a small dessert daily, or during their eating periods, but they make sure to take into consideration that it must be included in their calories.

A common mistake that people make is that they forget that what they are drinking also contains calories. Many people enjoy a good coffee beverage but fail to realize how much sugar is in the drink they order from a coffee shop. The same can be said for sodas, teas, and alcoholic beverages. So, make sure to do some research and find out how many calories are in the things you drink and add them to your caloric intake. Also, some people believe that avoiding all alcohol is best, but some people disagree. This is personal preference, but either way, you must know the calorie consumption and try not to go overboard.

Many people have their own guilty pleasures when it comes to what foods they crave. Intermittent fasting allows you to still indulge, while other diets might cut out foods completely. All you have to do is include the foods you love into the calories that you are consuming and stay within the limit. Of course, this might mean having smaller meals, but sometimes that indulgence means more simply because it can better your mental state. So, if a slice of chocolate cake is something you want, know you might have to make other sacrifices for it in reference to calories, but you can still eat the cake.

Sometimes foods just make us happy because we love them. Of course, there are some people out there who do not really feel this way, but for those people that do, being able to satisfy their craving is incredibly important to them. That is one of the reasons so many people choose intermittent fasting, because it doesn't make them give up the foods they love. It instead teaches them that they can still have it, just some adjustments to the rest of the day's food will need to be made. For so many people, that is a more than fair trade-off and one that they would be happy to make.

Changes Can Be Made

If you are doing the Crescendo method and end your eating period at 5:00 p.m. but find that you are incredibly hungry at 7:00 p.m., simply switch the times so you can allow yourself a small, last snack around 7:00 p.m. You have the power to do that. It might mean that you fast a little longer during the day, but if it works better with your body, then make the necessary changes. The same can be said if you are hungrier early in the morning, simply start your eating period earlier and end it earlier in the day. Some people simply prefer to eat more in the morning and some later in the day. Listen to your body and adjust the times to find what fits best into your lifestyle. Again, this also goes for people with less traditional hours, such as those who work third shift. If you find that you need to eat more late at night before you go to work and less in the morning before you get home and go to sleep, feel free to change your fasting period to accommodate that.

If you want faster, more drastic results, you can also change your eating habits completely, choosing to avoid simple or empty carbohydrates altogether. That's why people who practice the paleo or other keto diets can also benefit from intermittent fasting. If you do choose to do this, try to ease into it. You are already making one big lifestyle change, and to increase your chances of success, change your eating habits slowly. For instance, first just eliminate white bread and pasta from your diet and substitute wheat. Instead of eating a fast food burger, make one at home and use a wheat bun. These are rather small changes that can lead to big results. One of the best forms of motivation is seeing the results of your hard work. Making these changes will lead to the positive changes you want to see which in turn will only want to make you continue.

Some people find that it is also easier to begin their eating period in the middle of the day, so they have time to eat at work and at home. This is especially important for those people who want to save money since this gives them the opportunity to both bring their own lunch and cook their own dinner. Groceries are cheaper than getting takeout and going to a restaurant.

Cooking your own food and meal prepping also allows you to easily calculate how many calories you are consuming because you know exactly what is going into each meal.

Fixing Your Times

Some people might find that when doing the 5:2 method, including a weekend day as a fasting period, works best for them because they have that day off work completely. They can use this time to relax and find it easier to not eat when they have less obligations. Other people might find that having a weekend day as a fasting period ruins their weekend, because that is the time when they would rather go out with friends and being able to eat is important to them during that time.

There is absolutely nothing wrong with switching the days around if your first attempt didn't work out for you. Just simply switch the days until you do find a schedule that works for you. Just remember, you cannot fast for two consecutive days, so make sure to give yourself some time in between to refuel and give your body time to process what you have consumed. Your goal is to burn not only what you have recently eaten, but also some of the fat stores on your body, so take that into consideration also when you are making your fasting schedule.

Fasting on days when you are particularly active works for some because they find that it is easier to keep food off their minds when they have so many other things to focus on. Others find that fasting on these days is more difficult because they are just hungrier after doing so much. You don't want your body to feel exhausted and hungry all the time, so if you feel this way, it's time to reevaluate your schedule. Sit down and write out your normal plans for the week and try to schedule your fasting periods on the days when you are not as active. Doing this will make it easier on you and make your body feel better as well. The same goes for the reverse. If you think it would be easier to fast on days when you are more busy and you currently have your fasting period during your more less active times, switch it around. This cannot be stressed enough. Everyone is different and finding what works for you is the most important part of the process.

Sometimes a great place to start is asking yourself which is the most important meal of the day to you, it can be different for everyone. Once you know your answer, you can schedule your eating period to include that meal. If you are doing the 5:2 method, then you can also make that meal the heaviest in calories so you don't feel deprived of your favorite or most important meal. By doing this, you are not only going to feel better physically, but also mentally. Most people don't realize that it is not only the food that makes us happy, but also the ways in which we eat it. The example used earlier was preparing coffee in the morning. For some people, it is what helps them start their day, and going without the caffeine and traditional ritual can have detrimental effects to their mental state. That is what you want to avoid during a fast. If preparing an elaborate dinner is what makes you feel like you have a calm and relaxing end to your day, do not deny yourself of this, simply make it a priority when it comes to your fasting schedule.

This is not going to be an easy journey, especially in the beginning, but you can do it. Patience is key. Give both your mind and body time to adapt to this new schedule you are putting into place. Our bodies know how to burn fuel, and it can adjust to burning fat stores when needed, as long as it does not feel as though it is in starvation mode. Following the methods and sticking to the schedule will prevent this from happening and provide you with the results you want. If you have been sticking to your fasting schedule and are not seeing the results you wanted, you also have the option of eating cleaner or cutting out carbs. There are so many ways to tweak intermittent fasting to make it work for everyone.

Chapter 3: Fasting is On a Schedule, Use it to Save Money

The beauty of intermittent fasting is that you can decide when your fasting periods begin and end so there are no surprises. The same can't be said for other diets that require you to count calories or cut out all carbs. Having a set schedule makes it easy to plan your meals around your fasting periods, and no matter what type of method you are using, you can also meal plan or even take it a step further and meal prep to take all the guessing out of what you are going to eat, saving yourself even more money. In general, though, fasting means you are going to be eating less in general, so either way, you are going to save money.

It's no surprise that cooking at home is cheaper than going to restaurants, if done right, it can also be a lot healthier too. Food and restaurant advertising can feel overwhelming and make you feel that near constant eating is normal. That, of course, is not true. The human body is not built to eat all the time. Our culture is not also based around intermittent fasting either, so this is going to be one of the times in your life when you are going against the grain. Even though this can seem daunting, there is a level of freedom in knowing that you are paving your own way and listening to what your body is telling you, instead of doing what you think you should be doing. Many people are going to assume that you are starving yourself for a certain amount of time and some might caution or give you flack for your 'diet' choice. Remember, this is not a diet, this is a lifestyle and you already fast for a certain number of hours when you sleep. You are simply taking more control of your eating and fasting periods which helps you lose weight, gain mental clarity, and increase focus.

For most people who are trying to lose weight by using intermittent fasting, they treat it as a way for them to eat what they want, just not too much of it. Believe it or not, there is a connection between the way you spend money and the way you consume food. This connection is less based on the financial, and tends to actually have more emotional, almost irrational parallel. For instance, buying or ordering more than what you actually need. Many people find that when checking their bank account history, their food spending mirrored that of their emotional state at the time; it could peak and fall corresponding to someone's mood. This is the opposite of a schedule, and as things tend to be when led by emotion, unpredictable and in the case of food, more expensive than it needs to be.

Some of the common reasons people eat more than they need to can be connected to boredom, negative emotions, stress, or simply because they feel as though they need to. Intermittent fasting helps to end this way of thinking. Intermittent fasting allows you to treat eating as a chance to refuel, to let your body process and digest not only your last meal, but also fat stores. If you find yourself as an emotional or stress eater, then intermittent fasting is really going to benefit you.

Sometimes, we trick ourselves into thinking we need something when we actually don't, and in terms of food, this is not good for the body or the wallet. Think of intermittent fasting as giving yourself a new perspective. You are now going to think in terms of what you actually need and not what you want. Taking away the emotional aspect and replacing it with a strict schedule and foods that you need, is definitely going to cause some discomfort, but it will definitely be worth it. When you begin your chosen method of intermittent fasting, try to think about what you are getting, and not what you are missing. This definitely sounds easier said than done, but you are still going to be able to have moments of indulgence. There are just going to be fewer of them, and your body will thank you for it.

For those who are already on a tight budget and think that intermittent fasting is going to be too expensive, that couldn't be further from the truth. You are consuming fewer calories while intermittent fasting, meaning you are eating less, which in turn means you spend less on what you do eat. People have different reasons for intermittent fasting, and finding out why you are doing it and what you want to get out of it is going to help you succeed. So, start off by making a list of what you want to achieve through intermittent fasting as it will help you decide what you want to eat. Some people do not want to cook at home. For those people, it is still possible to save money because they too are going to go longer periods of time without eating.

If you do decide to most of your eating from restaurants, start asking how many calories are in the meals you eat. This is especially important if you are on the 5:2 method, because you do have strict limits for two days of the week. If you don't stick to the method of your choice, then you will not see any benefits, and not paying attention to the amount of calories that are in the foods you eat, you are going to set yourself back.

A New Schedule

Even though you probably think that you are going to be miserable from not eating, you will quickly find out that it is not the case. Intermittent fasting allows you to simplify your life. Think about how much time you spend, not just eating, but thinking about what to eat. Going longer times without eating means less stress and time spent worrying about what to eat. Many people are surprised by how much time went into food related matters and are amazed how much time is freed up when they begin their intermittent fasting lifestyle.

It is this newly acquired free time that gives you the freedom to accomplish more, it's almost like your days get longer. Suddenly, you have more time during the day to get work done, exercise, or simply relax. When you first begin your fasting method, it is a good idea to occupy your free time by keeping busy. There is definitely an adjust period, and it can be uncomfortable adapting to a new eating period. If you keep yourself busy, it can help keep your mind off of the fact that you might be hungry when your fasting period begins. This is one of the reasons so many people who practice intermittent fasting also take time to create a detailed grocery list to further reduce food related stress, and as yet another way to just simplify their lives.

You are probably going to notice an increase in your focus, discipline, and overall productivity. That is another one of the reasons people choose to change their lifestyle to include intermittent fasting. How people experience this varies from person to person. For instance, some people claim that they have more alertness in during the day when they skip breakfast and do not start their eating period until later in the day. While some people experience this later in the day, when their eating period has ended. Once you know how your body is going to react to this, you can schedule your important or major events or meetings to correspond with the times in which you feel more focused and alert.

Intermittent fasting requires a level of discipline that you might not have anticipated. This is part of the adjustment process and you will find that your overall discipline will also rise. This generally happens naturally, because you are retraining your brain to act and respond in a different way than it had previously. When you start to make more aware, careful decisions about food, it will simply translate to other aspects of your life. It feels nice to be in control, and intermittent fasting will show you that.

It is in your best interest to set yourself up for success. It is human nature to want to eat foods high in sugars and carbohydrates when your eating period beings after a long period of fasting. Again, it takes a lot of discipline to fast, but it takes even more discipline to eat completely clean and intermittent fast. That's why it is better for your mental health to allow for some indulgences from time to time. Part of setting up success means shopping ahead of time and knowing what you are going to put into your body and when. If your cupboards and refrigerator are full of healthy foods, then that is what you will eat when your fasting period ends.

The same can be said for self-sabotage. Since intermittent fasting does require self-discipline, it can be easy to accidentally overdo it with the calories. Of course, this doesn't mean that you need to eat clean all the time, but it does mean that you need put forth the effort to find out how many calories are in what you're eating. Some of the ways to help you prevent this from happening are to spread meals and snacks out during your eating period if your body responds better to that type of diet. If your body responds to two larger meals to feel satiated, then you can do it that way too. It's important to listen to your body and make changes accordingly.

Learning to listen to your body is one of the hardest parts of intermittent fasting since many people are accustomed to eating when they feel like it or when others are eating. So much of our lives revolve around food that many people have stopped listening to their bodies and started listening to what is around them, regardless of if they are actually hungry or not. This is a hard habit to break. One of the easiest places to start is to grocery shop when you are not hungry. This seems like common sense, but even people who are not intermittent fasting make this mistake. When you shop while hungry, you are more likely to throw unhealthy and over processed food into your cart because that is what you're craving at the moment.

Not only will this hurt your body, but it will also be harder on your wallet. Shopping smart doesn't just involve not shopping while hungry, it also means having a general idea of what you are going to buy before you go. This will make it easier to make healthy choices. Some people choose to meal plan or prep and make the same things each week, but this just personal preference and not something that you have to do, it is completely up to you. Finding what works for you can also be fun, try not to be too hard on yourself. You are making a lifestyle change. That means that you still need to live your life. Finding your stride and balance between fasting and living your life will happen, it just takes time and patience.

As you start your fasting journey remember to listen to your body. For some people, it has been a long time since they have done this in terms of food. However, this is the best way to ensure your success. Your body can and will tell you what it needs. That doesn't mean your body won't fight you when it is adapting to this new schedule of eating, but with time and discipline, both your mind and body will adapt, and you will reap the benefits. The unknown is scary for many people, so is intermittent fasting, because it is something they have not done previously. This is common and fortunately, it is short lived since intermittent fasting is not what many people expect, and the body is capable of more than what many people ask of it.

Chapter 4: Caloric Intake and Fasting

Many diets require you to reduce the amount of calories you consume by only allowing you to eat certain food. Granted, you are going to lose weight if you restrict calories, but you might also be miserable by doing so since you can't eat the foods you love. Even if you don't want to admit it, there are some foods that just make you feel better, whether it be chocolate cake or macaroni and cheese. You are only human, and there is nothing wrong with enjoying your food. Some diets make it nearly impossible to enjoy the foods you love, but intermittent fasting is not one of them.

It is simple math: if you reduce the calories you consume and still exercise the same amount or more than before, you will lose weight. Intermittent fasting reduces caloric intake by reducing the amount of time you are able to eat. It isn't that you are eating smaller meals or cutting out sugar or carbohydrates altogether, instead you are skipping meals completely and in doing so reducing your caloric intake. It's simple really, not eating for longer period of time means the hard work is done for you. No food was consumed, therefore your daily and weekly calorie count is lower.

Intermittent fasting is actually one of the least complex eating methods, which is one of the reasons it has gained so much in popularity. The beauty is in its simplicity. There are no points to keep track of, no carbohydrates to cut out, unless of course, you choose to. You probably think that you will want to binge once you begin your eating period after fasting, and at first you might, but this will change with just a little bit of time and discipline. Each method of fasting requires you to consume a healthy 2,000 calories during normal eating periods, and either no calories or very little during other times.

What you decide to eat during your eating period is up to you, but if you want the best results, choosing to fill those 2,000 calories with healthy, whole foods is going give you faster, more drastic results. Either way though, intermittent fasting still reduces stomach fat, and will only do it better and more quickly if you do decide to eat healthier. A flat stomach has more to do with what you eat and less to do with exercise. People are often surprised to hear this, but it is especially true for women. That's why intermittent fasting reduces stomach fat so quickly, because this is the type of food that begins with the food and a caloric deficit will show in stomach weight first for most women.

As long as you stick to your chosen method and do not exceed the 2,000 calories, you will automatically achieve a caloric deficit, which is the key to losing weight. Skipping entire meals reduces the amount of calories you eat, so much that you don't really have to worry too much about the calories you do eat when your fasting period is over. For example, if you eat peanut butter, toast, and a glass of orange juice in the morning, this by itself is around 500 calories. Some people also have a morning or midmorning tea or coffee beverage that can contain up to 150 calories, for instance, the average latte contains around 130. If you were to fast in the morning and not start eating until around lunch time, you are cutting out nearly 700 calories.

If a woman eats between 1,600 to 2,000 calories per day, just skipping that one meal is between twenty to almost thirty percent of their caloric intake saved instantly. Then, later in the day, if you ate two larger meals that are around 750 calories each, and a dessert around 300 calories, you are still only consuming 1,800 calories which is well on the way to weight loss. Even better is that you do not have to give up anything that you love. This is about changing the times that you eat, not what you eat.

Intermittent fasting is also one of the easiest ways to burn actual fat. For instance, when you start a low carbohydrate diet, the number on the scale will drop quickly, but you are losing water from your body, not real fat. Sometimes, you can also cut calories so much that the body will actually hold onto fat cells and burn muscle as an alternative source of fuel. This is what happens when the body goes into starvation mode, and that is what you want to avoid. Intermittent fasting, when done properly, will not cause you to lose muscle mass. Your body will not feel like it is going into starvation and will burn fat stores to use as energy. This is how you lose weight and keep it off.

If you find yourself losing muscle mass or not seeing the desired results, you can and should tweak your fasting times or caloric intake. As mentioned before, the best way to gauge this is to listen to your body. There are different types of intermittent fasting for a reason. Not everyone is built the same and everyone's body responds differently. That's why you can change the times to match what works for you. Just make sure not to go too far above an average healthy caloric intake, or too far below it either, since that can be just as harmful. The key is to be patient and listen to your body, but don't be too strict, this isn't meant to make you miserable and moody, which can happen if you aren't being safe.

What you put into your body when you do eat is completely your choice. As you have seen, skipping meals already gives you an edge with the caloric deficit, but you can take it a step further and choose to eat very healthy when your eating period begins. Of course, this is not going to be easy as the body is going to feel run down and craving foods rich in carbohydrates and sugar. However, you can eat a lot more vegetables and fruits than sugary and carbohydrate heavy foods, meaning you will feel fuller while eating less calories. Some people choose to do this because it frees them up to have more snacks during their eating period or allows them to have a more calorie heavy dessert.

You also have to remember that it is important to burn calories too, and in the beginning the last thing you are going to want to do is exercise, especially during your fasting period. That is perfectly fine. It is actually recommended to do light exercise while fasting, but some people prefer to do heavier workouts during a fasting period. Only do what your body can handle, there is no one right way to fast intermittently. What works for one person might not work for another. The same goes for exercising and fasting, it might take some trial and error before you figure out what works well for you. Some people try to keep up with their regular exercise routines but find that it is too intense during their fasting period. If you feel this way, lighten up your workout on fasting days if you are doing the 5:2 or eat-stop-eat method. If you are doing any of the other methods, you can learn to plan your workouts around your food intake times.

One of the most common things that people do is to plan their eating times around their workouts, or vice versa. After a workout the body is typically very hungry, and hard workouts and fasting can be a recipe for failure. You can prevent this from happening by working out based on your eating period. Exercise when you still have time to eat afterwards if that is how your body operates. On the other hand, if your body works better with a larger meal before a heavy workout, cater to it that way.

Most people plan their food out based on how it makes them feel in terms of their energy levels throughout the day, which includes their exercise routine. They want to feel their best which serves as natural motivation to eat healthier, because it keeps them from feeling sluggish during the day and lets them workout harder. Generally, this comes with time and experience, because everyone is different. Some people might find that they prefer to eat a high carbohydrate vegetarian diet, while others prefer a low carbohydrate, but higher fat and protein diet to feel their best. Eat when and what works for you but be consistent. Your diet and fast doesn't have to match someone else's, but you won't see the results and reap the benefits of intermittent fasting if you are not consistent with what works for you.

If you are doing the eat-stop-eat method, then you are going a full 24 hours without eating, two to three times each week. For fasts that are long like that, it is a good idea to use those days to do light exercise or as resting days. If you do choose to do some form of exercise on these days, begin with some light exercises to see how your body responds before you jump into a heavier workout. A good example of some exercises to do include: yoga, speed walking, swimming, and anything else that is relatively low impact. If you do not feel light headed or dizzy from this, continue to increase your workouts until you see fit, as long as you stop if you feel any detrimental side-effects of the workouts.

You do not have to stick to the 2,000 calories a day either, you can safely drop to 1,600 as that is a healthy amount too. The 2,000 calorie is an average, and for those who are trying to lose weight, it would be more beneficial for them to stick to a 1,600 calorie a day diet. You can always adjust your caloric intake as you go depending on the results you are seeing. It's helpful to also know that once you reach a healthy weight, your body will naturally maintain it and weight loss will slow down. This usually happens after a year or so of intermittent fasting, and one of the reasons it is so effective is because it takes very little to maintain a healthy weight. It is also another reason that intermittent fasting is considered a lifestyle and not a diet, because once you have made it a habit, it feels natural and becomes your new normal.

Just remember that intermittent fasting is not meant to feel like torture, of course it is going to take some time to adjust to, but if after a few weeks you feel tired and rundown, make some changes. You have the power to change nearly everything about how you fast, as long as you follow the basic rules and always take your safety into consideration. You do not have to give up the chocolate you love so much, or not train for the marathon you've been looking forward to. In fact, you can still eat what you want, exercise normally, and still manage to either lose weight or maintain a healthy weight.

The hardest part of this journey is going to be the beginning. Many people find they don't really know where to start, or how to begin. There is no secret, you just have to do it. That's it. Sure, you might stumble or break your fast before you're supposed to sometimes, but just try again the next day and make changes if you feel you need to. Your body knows what it's doing, it's your job to listen to it, and intermittent fasting is a great way to learn to do that. So, don't be afraid to make some mistakes, it's the best way to learn sometimes. You need to know what not to do to find what works for you sometimes, and that's okay.

Chapter 5: Save Money, Make a Grocery List

You already know that you are going to be eating less, an entire meal is going to be left out of your diet. That means that you get to spend less at the grocery store too. For instance, if you begin your eating period around lunch and continue through dinner, that means that you are not eating breakfast. Consider, it a thing of the past. Not only is it something that you don't have to worry about anymore, but it's also something that you don't have to pay for anymore either. This frees you up to just buy lunch, dinner, snack, and dessert foods, most of which are interchangeable. Of course, the exception to this is the 5:2 and the eat-stop-eat methods where you are eating all three meals on other days, but significantly cutting calories on the other two days, or fasting altogether.

Regardless of the method that you chose, the best thing you can do to save money is to cook at home and meal prep. Not only does this reduce the stress of wondering what you are going to eat, it also means that you can make a plan which will help you make better choices. Of course, you do not have to do it this way, but it can really help to simplify your life and get the most benefits from intermittent fasting. You are probably thinking about how much more expensive it is to eat healthier foods, when processed, prepackaged, or takeout is so much cheaper. Well, sometimes that may be true, there are some things that you can do to eat healthier even on the super tight budget.

Tips to Shopping on a Budget – And Keep It Healthy

- Work with your environment and the season. Fruits and vegetables that are in season are cheaper than their counterparts that are transported from farther away. So, feel free to stock up on the cheaper fruits and veggies and then freeze them to use later. Make sure to label everything with the date and check to see how long it will keep when frozen, since some items keep longer than others. You can also prep smoothies in this way too, so all you have to do is throw them in the blender with some yogurt or milk if you prefer for a healthy snack or dessert.

- Shop smart. If your grocery store or co-op has a member card that gives discounts, get it. Also, check the circulars and shop what is on sale. This will be a great way to create variety since sales change so often. One of the best ways to save money is to be buy the protein that is on sale that week and plan your meals around that. You might be eating a lot of fish or chicken in one week, but it will be cheaper than going out or not buying what it is on sale. Plus, it can be a fun way to learn to cook things you didn't know how to before. The internet is a wonderful place to find healthy recipes. It doesn't matter if you are vegan or meat eater, you can find something interesting to make with the ingredients that are on sale.

- Speaking of meat, get a little adventurous with the cuts that you get. Obviously, some are more expensive than others, so go with a cheaper cut. You are intermittent fasting after all, consuming less calories is par for the course. You can add a little bit of a fattier cut of meat into your diet. Also, bone-in, tougher cuts, and skin-on cuts are all going to be cheaper. If you are feeling even more adventurous, organs are also incredibly cheap and are nutritious and flavorful. This is also another great opportunity to explore less traditional recipes online. Another great rule of thumb when it comes to tougher cuts of meat in general, don't forget to bring out the crockpot. Sometimes, that is the secret to making even the toughest cuts delicious and healthy.

- If you are vegan or vegetarian, you are no stranger to different types of beans and grains.

However, if it's new to you, learn to embrace whole grains and substitute beans for meat in your meals throughout the week. Beans are cheaper than meat and are also nutritious. Avoid white bread if you can, since it is empty carbohydrates and provides very little nutritional value and opt for the whole wheat bread that is on sale instead. Sometimes, there is a manager's special in the bakery department on breads that are a little older. So, don't forget to check there, and don't be shy to ask someone who works there if you can't find it easily. Other cheap grains are freekeh, brown rice, and quinoa.

- Explore foods from other cultures, for instance, Mexican food relies heavily on rice and beans. Use brown rice as a healthy and cheap alternative. Indian food is another flavorful and healthy option. If you think that you don't like Indian or Mexican food, look up different recipes online, chances are you just haven't found the right dish yet. Or it might not be the entire entrée that you don't like, but a specific herb or spice. An example is that, to some people, cilantro tastes like soap. So just keep trying until you find something you like. Don't be scared to tweak recipes that you find to make them more personally palatable.

- This should probably go without saying, but keep your kitchen organized. Know what ingredients you are out of, or running low on. It can be difficult to eat healthy after a day of long, hard work, only to come home and find out that you are out of chicken, or quinoa. That's when the temptation to order unhealthy takeout might win. This is another reason meal planning is so important; it will prevent issues like this from occurring. If you keep an organized kitchen and have a specific plan set out that includes everything you need to eat for the week, down to each ingredient, then the more likely you are to have everything and eat healthier.

- One of the greatest ways to save money is to reduce waste. You can do this by getting creative and repurposing your leftovers. Again, the internet is a wonderful place to find recipes for nearly anything. For instance, if you bake a chicken, you cannot only use the bones to create your own bone broth, but you can also use any of the leftover meat to make a soup or even a healthy wrap for lunch the next day. Don't throw food away if you think you can make something with it later. You can even freeze items if you think you can use them later.

- Shop at other places. There is no reason that you have to do all of your shopping at the same store unless you want to. Different stores are going to have different sales for you to take advantage of, and swing by your local farmer's market right before they close. Vendors are more likely to give you a good deal just so they don't have to transport it back and forth.

- Another option is bargaining, and bargain bins for ugly produce. These are the fruits and vegetables that are slightly bruised or nearly overripe. They are often highly discounted at stores. You can also ask the local farmer's market vendor to sell you their 'ugly' produce for cheaper. More often than not it gets thrown away, making your chances of getting it for cheap even higher.

- Check out your local ethnic markets too, you will be surprised what you find there at bargain prices. Also, you can find some interesting proteins, fruits, and vegetables too, usually at very reasonable prices. For instance, rice noodles in a traditional grocery store can be expensive, but at an Asian market they are much cheaper.

- Don't be afraid to try new things. Remember to keep an open mind when you are wondering around different places. Just because you haven't had something before, doesn't mean it's bad. It probably just means you are going to have to learn to prepare it properly and figure out how to work into your meal planning. Some of the best things come from happy accidents. Stumbling upon interesting and unique ingredients are no exception.

- The most important tip of all, again, try not to go grocery shopping while you're hungry. Your hunger is going to prevent you from making sound, healthy decisions, and if you have the power to prevent that, do it. If you have no other option, make a detailed list and try your best to stick it.

Meal prepping is going to be the easiest choice, since you can make a detailed grocery list mapping out everything you are going to eat or drink during the week. However, this method is not for everyone. For those people who hate to cook or who just prefer takeout and restaurants, there's nothing wrong with that as long as you also make healthy choices. The key to this is going to be communication. Act like you are shopping for your food and don't be shy about asking what ingredients are in the food you are ordering, as well as the calorie count. A good rule of thumb: if there is no way to determine how many calories are in an entrée, don't order it. You can always look things up online, but to do so accurately, you need to know the amount of the different ingredients.

It doesn't matter if you are shopping for yourself or ordering out, your goal is to make good decisions. When you prefer to not cook at home, it can take some creativity as well. For instance, get familiar with the ala carte menu at your favorite restaurants. The portions are generally listed, and you can look up your caloric intake online if you need to. Also, branch out, try different types of restaurants such as Turkish, Ethiopian, or even Vietnamese if you haven't had it before. There are a lot of new and fun healthy options out there. These types of restaurants can also be much cheaper too.

If you find that you are spending too much money from eating out, then you can do a combination of cooking at home and going out. Many people will meal plan and prep for the weekdays and allow their weekends to be a bit more spontaneous so they can go out with friends. If this is the method you choose, don't forget to check the calories. You need to have some idea, just so you know how much you can eat or drink later.

This brings us to adult beverages. Some people are going to say to abstain from them altogether, while others are going to say it's fine in moderation. Just be sure to add the calories from your drinks into your daily intake and avoid them altogether during fasting periods. This is completely personal preference. If you want to forgo dessert in favor of a glass of wine or a cocktail, do it. Again, not only is this your life, but your fast, and you are free to do as you please. Of course, remember that alcohol does have sugar in it and it is not going to help in weight loss. But knowing what you know, if you still want that glass of wine, make the necessary sacrifice other calories from something else and enjoy.

No matter which method you choose, or what you decide to eat, you are making a decision for yourself and taking your eating schedule into your own hands. It might not always be easy, but few things worth it ever are. Your hard work, dedication, and discipline will pay off in the end! So, just keep going, be patient with yourself, and learn from your mistakes. You're allowed to make mistakes and learn from them, it's part of the process when there is no one-size-fits-all fasting method. So, don't be too hard on yourself and remember to have some fun.

CPSIA information can be obtained
at www.ICGtesting.com
Printed in the USA
BVHW072313200421
605395BV00007B/1610

9 781087 849362